Chill Out

Practicing Calm

Reach Out!

Learning to overcome negative thoughts and stay mindful is not the same as fighting depression. Do you feel overwhelmed by sadness? Remember, you matter. You are not alone. If you need help, reach out. Talk to an adult you love and trust. This could be a teacher, school counselor, or family member. Make an appointment with your doctor. Seek professional help. Or call the National Suicide Prevention Lifeline at 1-800-273-8255. Someone is available to talk with you 24 hours a day, every day.

45th Parallel Press

Published in the United States of America by Cherry Lake Publishing
Ann Arbor, Michigan
www.cherrylakepublishing.com

Reading Adviser: Marla Conn, MS, Ed., Literacy specialist, Read-Ability, Inc.
Book Designer: Melinda Millward

Photo Credits: © Daisy Daisy/Shutterstock.com, back cover, 24; © Dean Drobot/Shutterstock.com, cover, 5; © DreamStockIcons/Shutterstock.com, 6; © roxxyphotos /stock.adobe.com, 7; © LUIS PADILLA-Fotografia/Shutterstock.com, 8; © Wavebreakmedia/istockphoto.com, 9;© MAKSIM ANKUDA/Shutterstock.com, 10; © ALEAIMAGE/istockphoto.com,11; © Kamenetskiy Konstantin/Shutterstock.com, 12; © kuroksta/Shutterstock.com, 14, 22; © Subbotina Anna/Shutterstock.com, 15; © Tetiana Rostopira/Shutterstock.com, 16; © Olkita/Shutterstock.com, 18; © simona /stock.adobe.com, 19; © Ollyy/Shutterstock.com, 20; © Rock and Wasp/Shutterstock.com, 21; © Supawadee56/Shutterstock.com, 23; © Viktorija Reuta/Shutterstock.com, 26; © Neustockimages/istockphoto.com, 27; © johnfoto18/Shutterstock.com, 28; © PHILIPIMAGE/Shutterstock.com, 30; © paranut/Shutterstock.com, 30

Graphic Element Credits: © kkoman/Shutterstock.com, back cover, front cover, multiple interior pages; © str33t cat/Shutterstock.com, front cover, multiple interior pages; © NotionPic/Shutterstock.com, multiple interior pages; © CARACOLLA/Shutterstock.com, multiple interior pages; © VikiVector/Shutterstock.com, multiple interior pages

45th Parallel Press is an imprint of Cherry Lake Publishing.

Library of Congress Cataloging-in-Publication Data has been filed and is available at catalog.loc.gov

Printed in the United States of America
Corporate Graphics

Table of Contents

INTRODUCTION

Have you ever felt overwhelmed? Are things out of control? Do you feel **stressed** out? Stress is the pressure that builds up inside you from difficult situations in life. It causes people to worry. People get tense. They get nervous. Stress stops people from doing things. It makes people feel helpless. It can make people **panic**. Panic means to feel sudden and extreme fear or worry.

It's important to relax. Learning to be calm will help you manage stress. It will quiet your mind. It will make you more peaceful.

This book gives you tips on how to be **mindful**. Mindful means being aware. It means taking care of your body and mind. Take a moment. Practice being calm. Just breathe …

Tip: Being calm can be hard sometimes. But if you practice every day, you'll get into the habit of being calm.

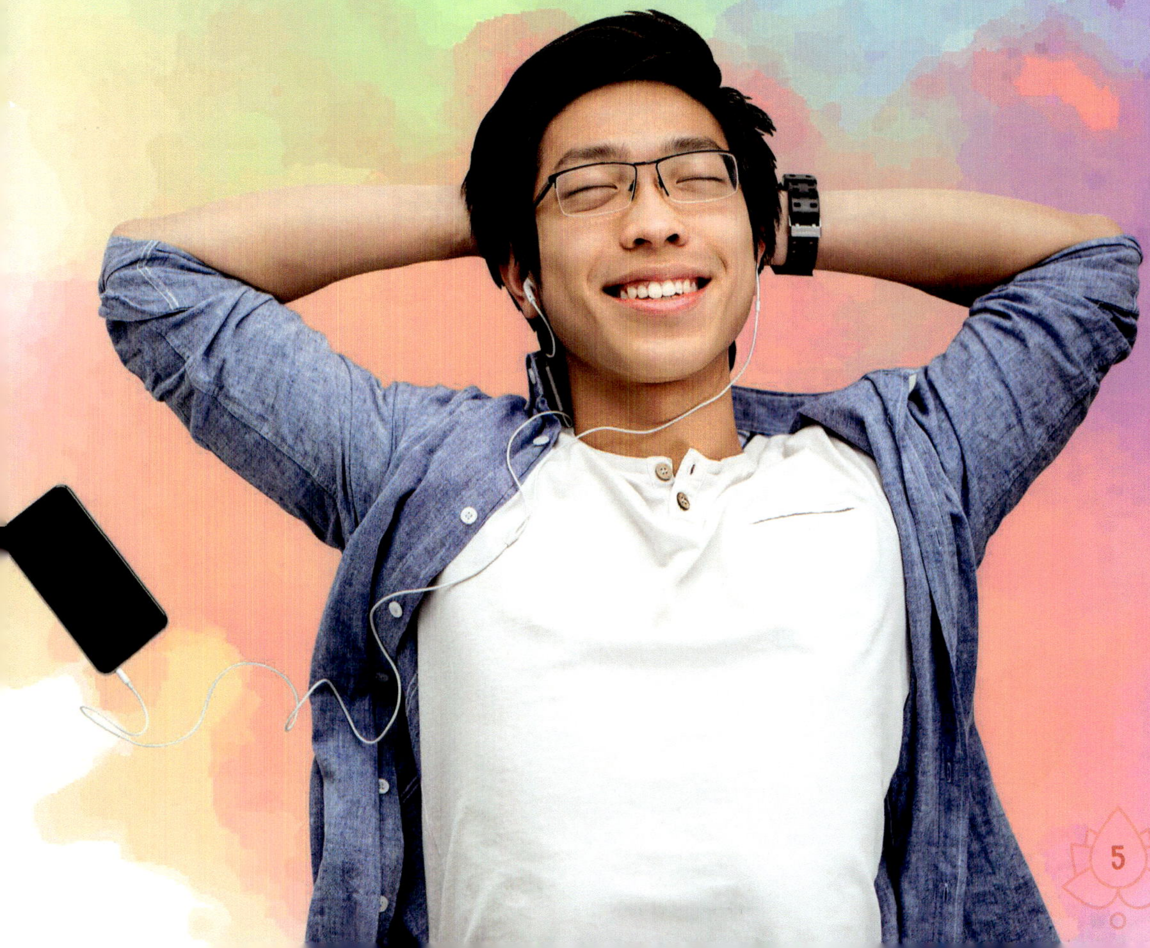

CHAPTER ONE
Count Your Breaths

Stress affects how we breathe. Our breathing becomes short. It becomes fast. Some people find it hard to breathe. When this happens, it's important to catch your breath. Get your breathing back to normal. Taking deep breaths is good for you. It's a quick and easy way to calm your nerves. There are many breathing activities.

One activity is called birthday candles. Hold up your hand. Stretch out your fingers. Pretend your fingers are candles. Count out the 5 candles. Blow out each candle with a long breath. Curl your finger down slowly while blowing.

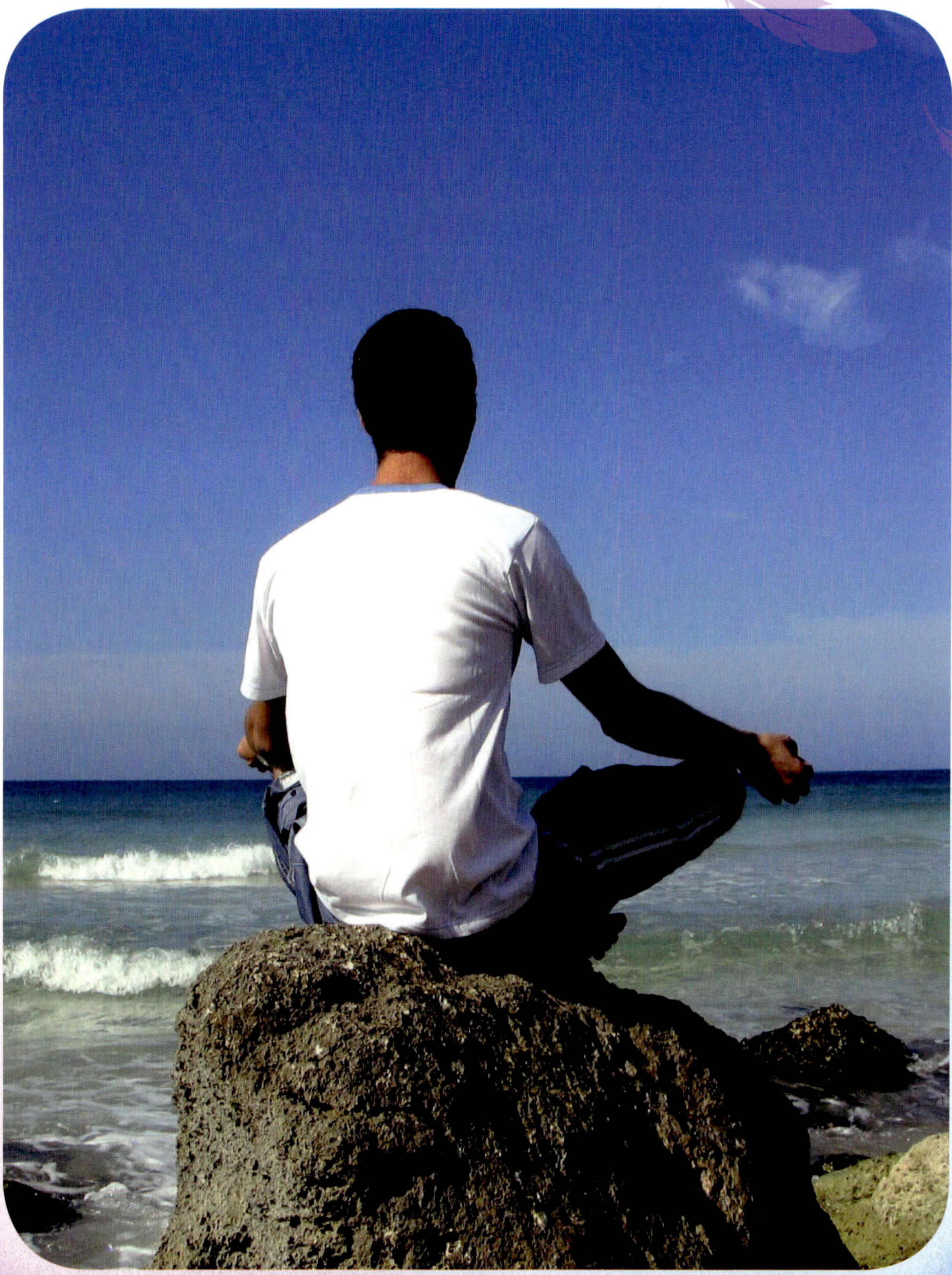

Tip: Count backward from 100.

Another activity is called balloons. Pretend to pull a balloon out of your pocket. Cup your hands together. Hold them in front of your mouth. Take a deep breath. Let go of your breath. Do this slowly. Open your hands as you blow. Pretend you're blowing up a balloon. When the balloon is full, take another deep breath. Slowly close your hands back together as you breathe in.

This next activity is called **pinwheel**. Pinwheels are sticks with colored wheels. The wheels twirl or spin in the wind. Get a pinwheel. Practice different types of breathing. Control your breath. Make the pinwheel go slow. Make it go fast. Make it stop and go.

Tip: Watch fish swim in a tank. Take deep breaths while you do this. Count your breaths.

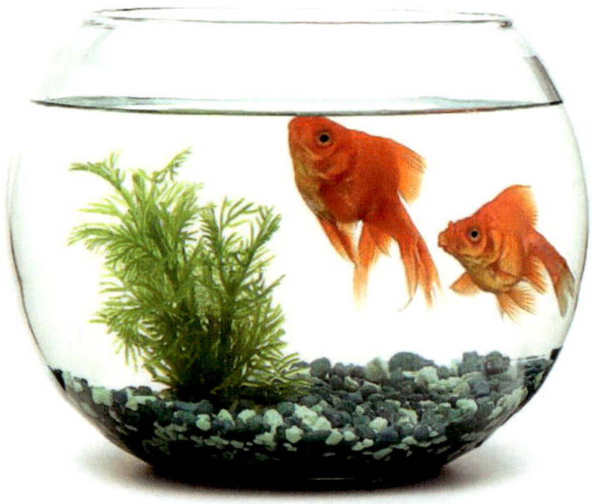

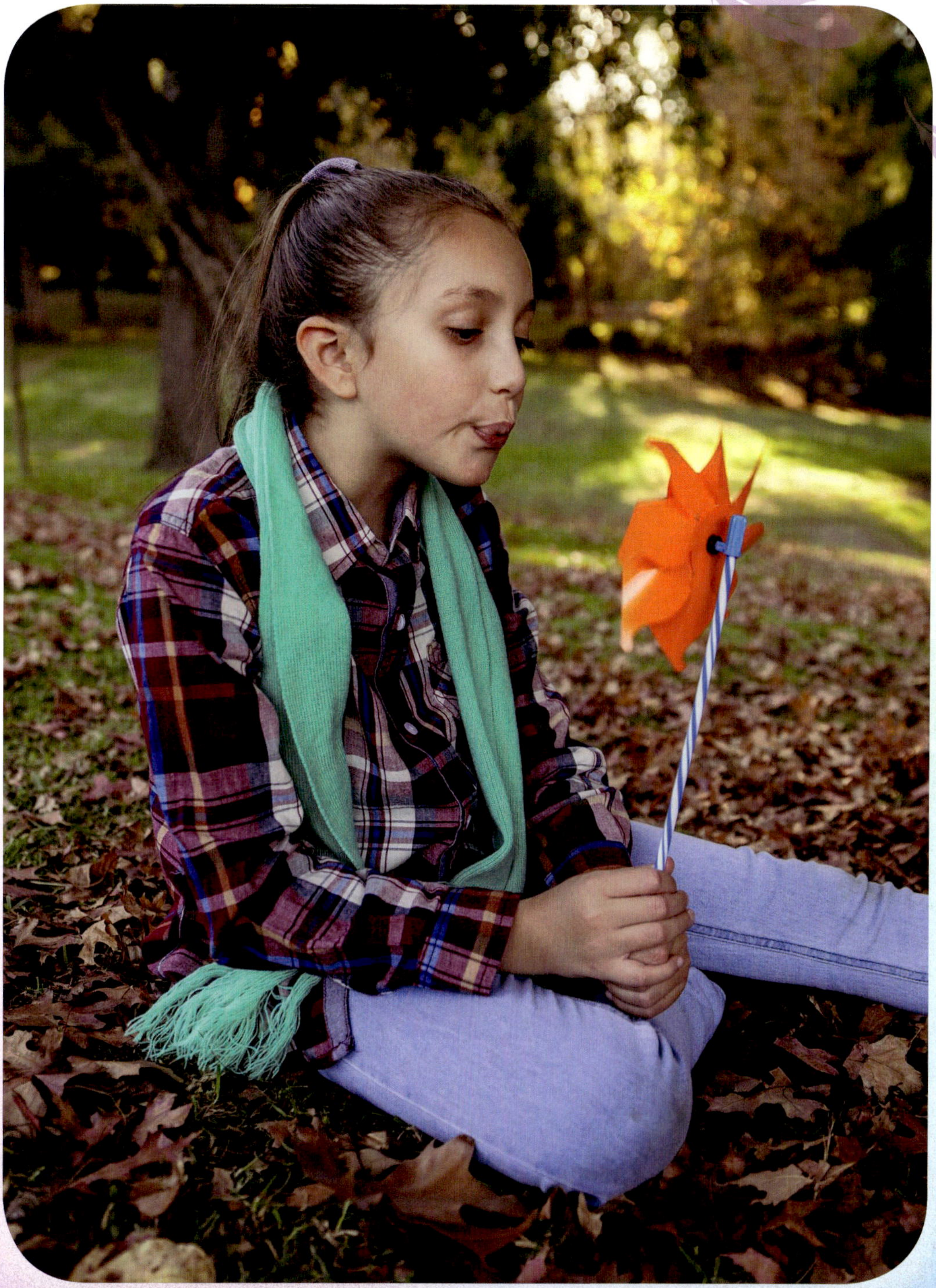

CHAPTER TWO
Relax Your Muscles

Stress makes the body tense up. It tightens muscles. Tight muscles cause aches and pains. This makes the body weak. Practice training your muscles. When your body is relaxed, you'll feel less **anxious**. Anxious means extreme worry. Find a comfortable place. Lie down on your back. Tighten and relax 1 muscle group at a time.

Take a deep breath in. As you do this, tighten a muscle group. Do this for about 10 seconds. Then, slowly breathe out. As you do this, relax your muscles. Relax for 10 to 20 seconds. Then, work on the next muscle group.

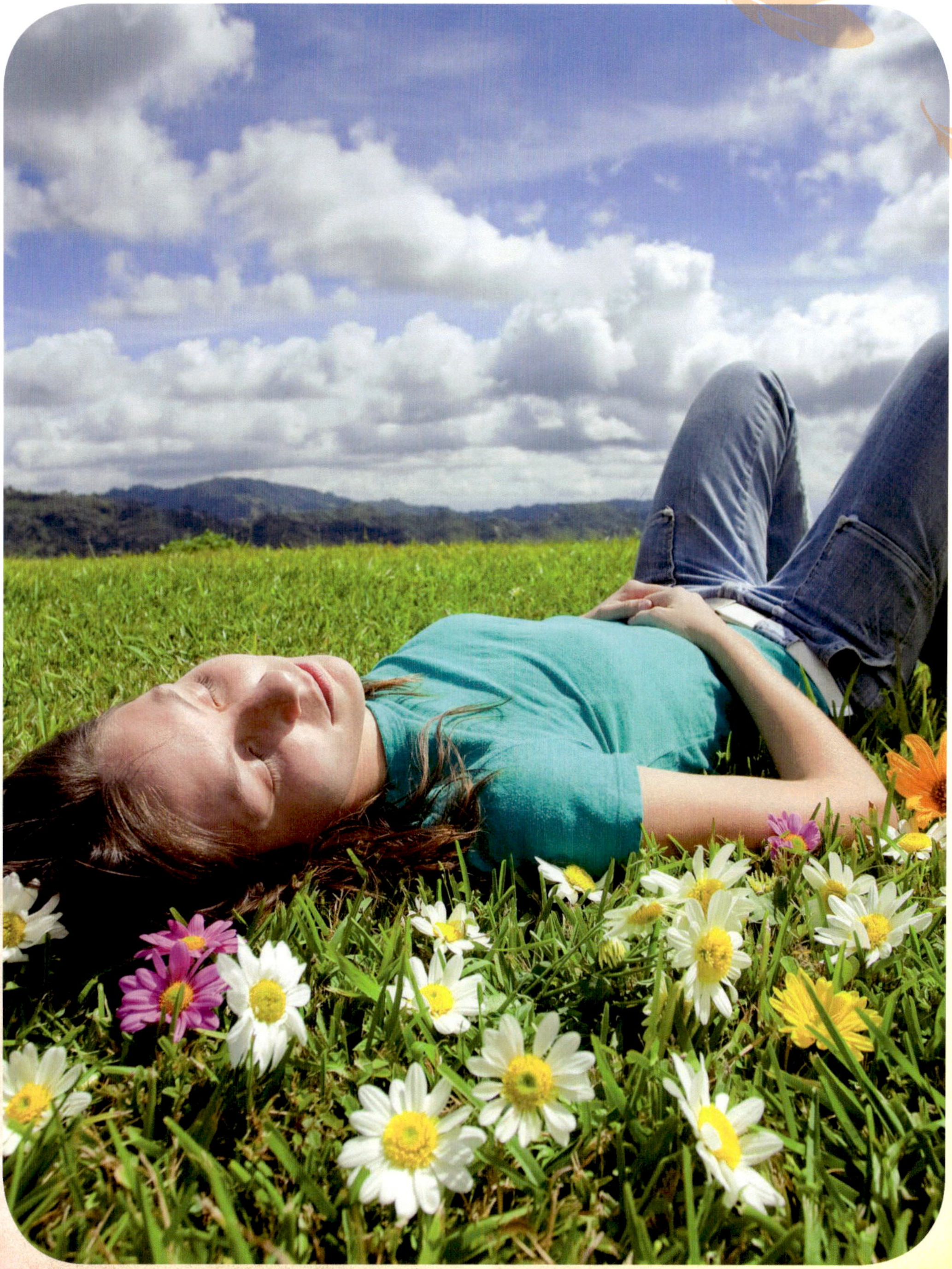

Tip: To sleep better, relax your muscles. Try taking a warm shower or bath before bed. The warm water will relax your muscles.

Work the muscle groups in this order:

- Make your hands into fists. Then, slowly release them.
- Raise your arms up in the air and reach out. Then, bring your arms down to your sides. Let them swing side to side.
- Lift your shoulders toward your ears. Rotate them forward and backward in tiny circles.
- Stand and bend at your waist. Let your head and arms fall heavy. Try to sway up and down, side to side. Slowly roll yourself up to standing.
- Suck your stomach into a tight knot. Push your stomach out. Then bring your stomach back to its normal resting position.
- While sitting, stretch out your legs. Tighten your thighs and calves. Slowly release them.
- Point your toes toward your face. Point your toes away. Curl them downward. Then release the tension and bring your toes back to rest.

Tip: Stretch your muscles. Touch your toes. Reach for the sky. Stretch out your arms and legs to form the letters of your name.

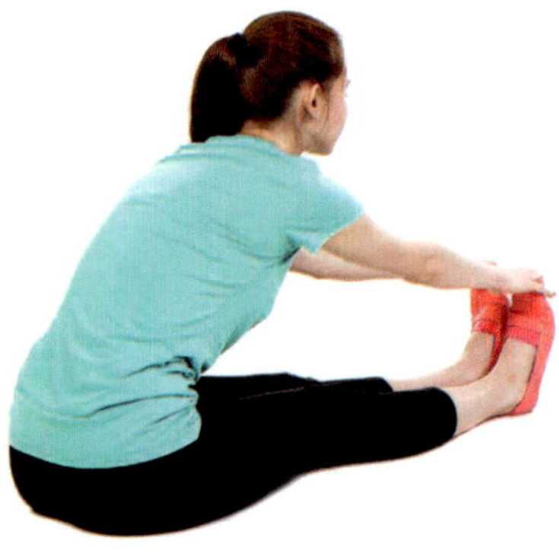

Real-Life Scenarios

Life is full of adventures. There will be challenges. Things happen. Make good choices. These are some events you could face:

- You have 3 tests in the same week. You also have to practice for a big game. Does this stress you out? Did you prepare? How are you going to manage your time?
- You found out your best friend was talking about you. You feel upset. Your body reacts. Your heart is racing. Your blood is boiling. What else do you feel? How can you best handle your feelings?
- You just got some bad news. You start to cry. You can't stop. The tears keep coming. You're having a hard time breathing. How can you calm yourself down? What can you do to feel better?

Chapter Three
Channel Your Energy

If you're nervous, you may have a lot of extra energy. This means you're restless. You can't sleep. You have a hard time staying still. You're feeling jittery. To calm yourself, you need to get rid of the energy.

Channel your energy. Channel means to guide or direct. Do something active. Do something creative.

You can work on a **hobby**. Hobbies are activities done for fun. These activities could be art, sports, or writing. Take your skills to another level. Push yourself. Tasks should be hard enough to be challenging. But if you find yourself getting frustrated, pause what you're doing. Take a break. Do something else. Then go back to the task.

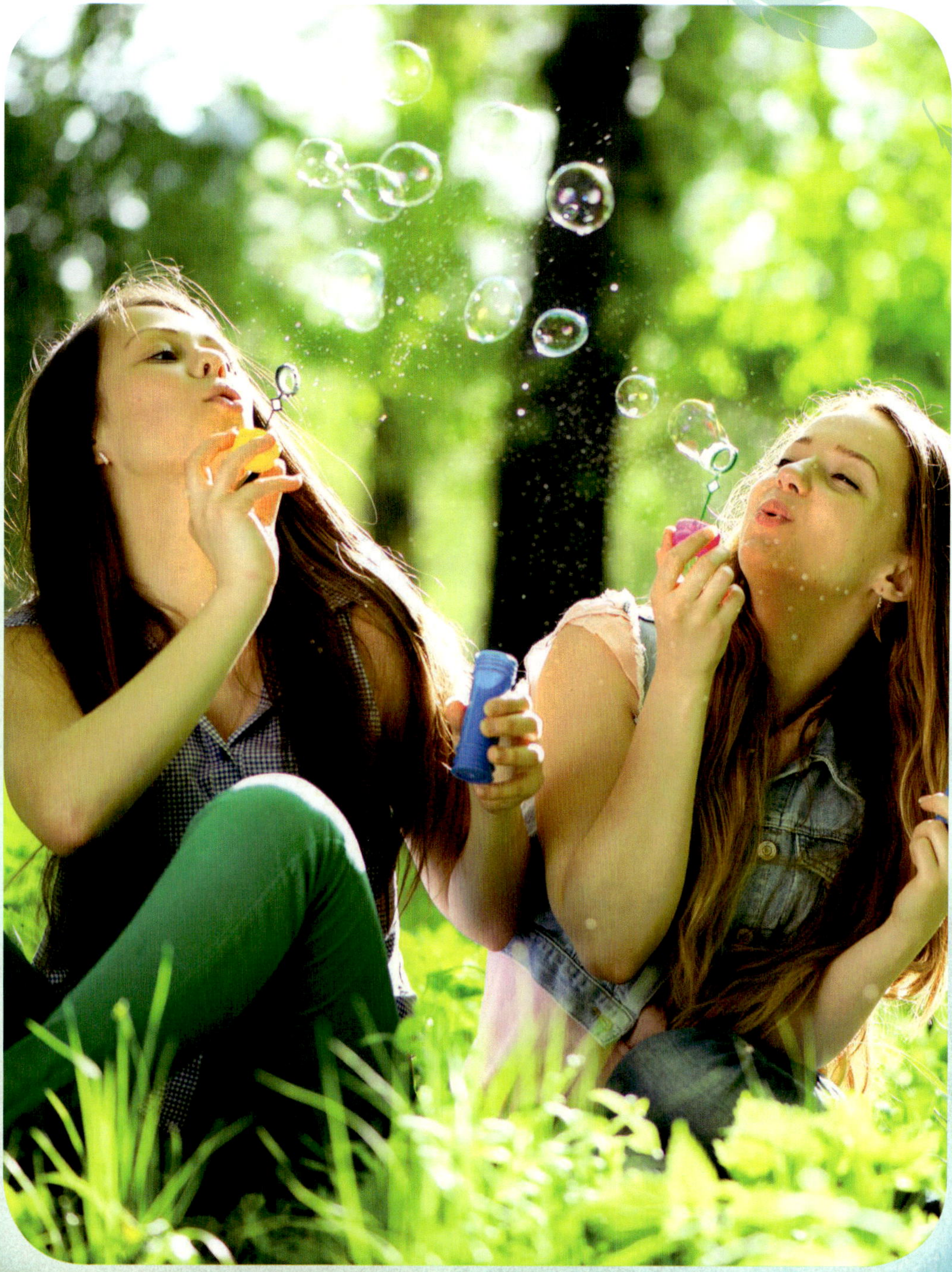

Tip: Blow bubbles. Imagine your worries are in the bubbles. Watch the bubbles float away. Watch them pop.

Some people enjoy **doodling**. Doodling means scribbling or drawing. Make doodle art. Use a black marker. Start at the corner of a paper. Make large loops. Cover the entire page. Make different loops and circles. Go in different directions. Don't stop until you're done with your doodle. Then color in the spaces. Use different colors for each space.

Some people enjoy coloring books. Try this tip to create light and dark colors. Use your favorite coloring book. Lightly color in a space. Add a drop of baby oil to a cotton swab. Rub the cotton swab over the color. Let the oil dry. This will create darker shades.

Tip: Jump rope or hula hoop. Being active can help release bad feelings.

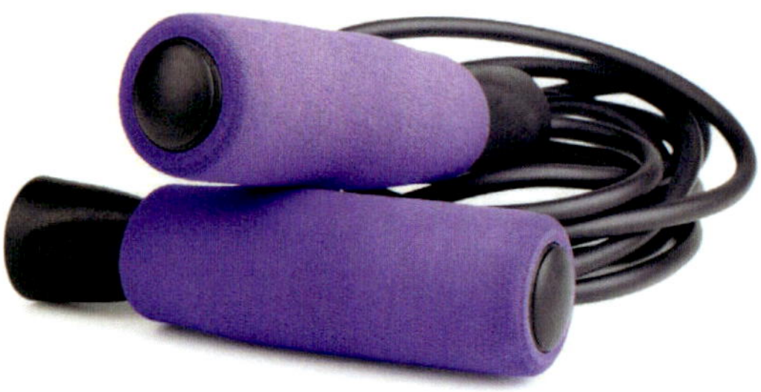

Science Connection

Stress affects your body. It makes you go into a fight-or-flight mode. This means you either want to fight or run away. Stress affects the brain. There's a small area in the base of the brain. It's called the hypothalamus. It releases bursts of energy in the body. It makes your heart and blood pump more. It makes your muscles tight. It makes you more hyper. Hyper means active. Stress is needed to deal with dangers. It helps keep us alive. It helps us survive. It also keeps us alert and focused. But too much stress is bad. Feeling stressed for a long time is also bad. Stress can cause aches and pains. It can make you sick. It can cause heart attacks. By calming down, the body balances itself.

CHAPTER FOUR
Engage Your Senses

Your **senses** might overload when you're feeling stressed. Senses include sight, sound, smell, taste, and touch. Lower your stress level by trying sensory activities.

Make touch bins. Get several shoe boxes. Fill each box with different things. Examples are sand, rice, and beans. Run your hands through the box. Let the items slip through your fingers. Keep doing this until you're calm.

Give yourself a foot **massage**. Massages are the rubbing of muscles to ease pain. There are pressure points on your feet. Applying different pressures to these points can help you relax. Roll a golf ball under your feet. Apply different pressures.

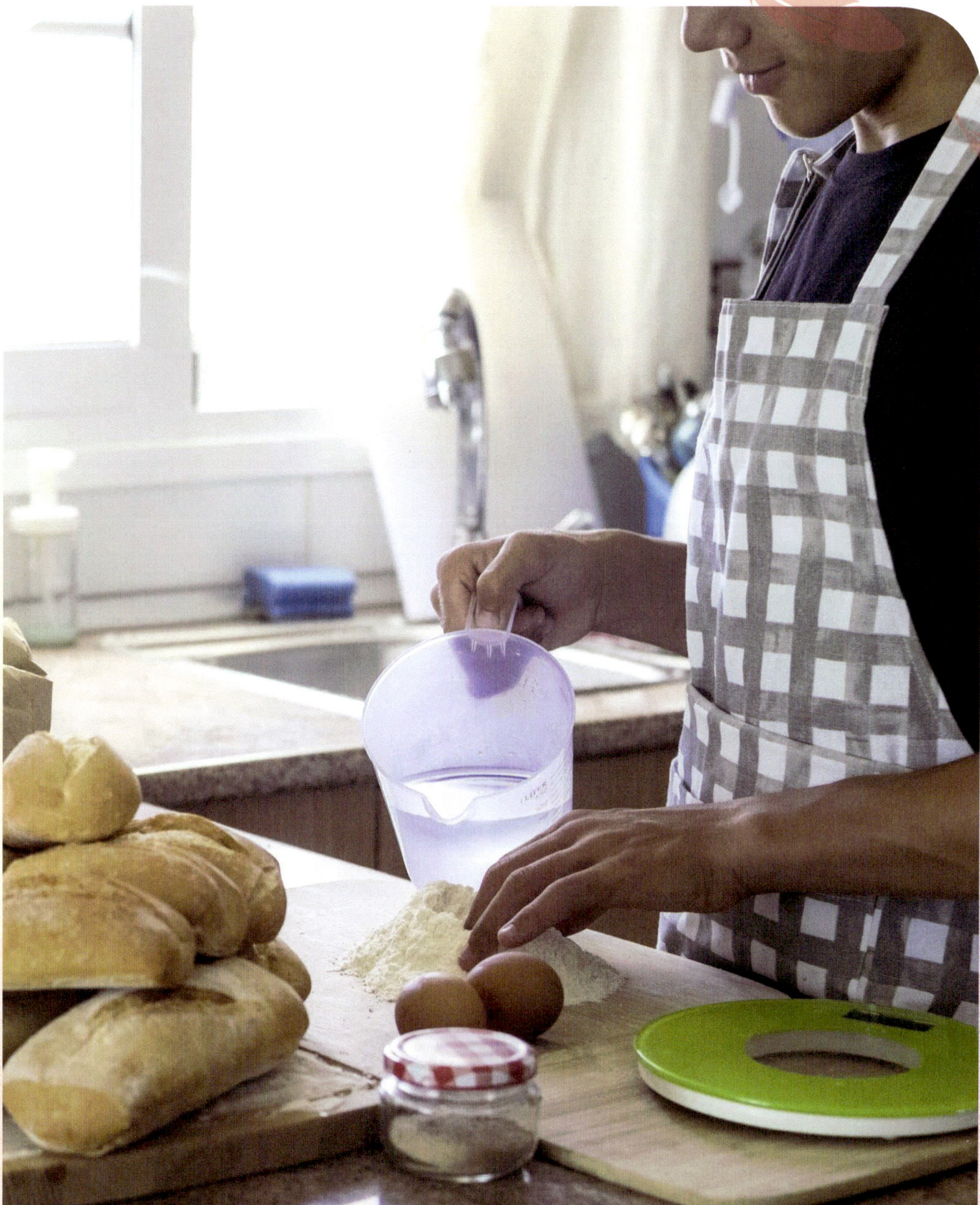

Tip: Make dough. Work the dough into different shapes. Think of the task as working out your worries.

Apply pressure to your body. You can do this by hugging someone. Hug for at least 20 seconds. You can also wrap yourself with a heavy blanket. You can sit in a beanbag chair.

Keeping your mouth busy can be calming. Blow a feather across a table. Chew gum. Suck a thick milkshake through a straw.

Make "calm down jars." Get a plastic or glass jar with a lid. Fill it with water and glitter. Shake the jar. Watch the glitter slowly move from the top of the jar to the bottom. Listen to music as you do this.

Play the "tea bag matching game." Get several different tea bags. Take the tea bags out of the wrappers. Cut off the tags. Make two piles. One with the tags and the other with the tea bags. Smell the tea in the bags. Match them with the tags.

Tip: Make a playlist of calming music. Listen to the songs. Clap your hands to the beat.

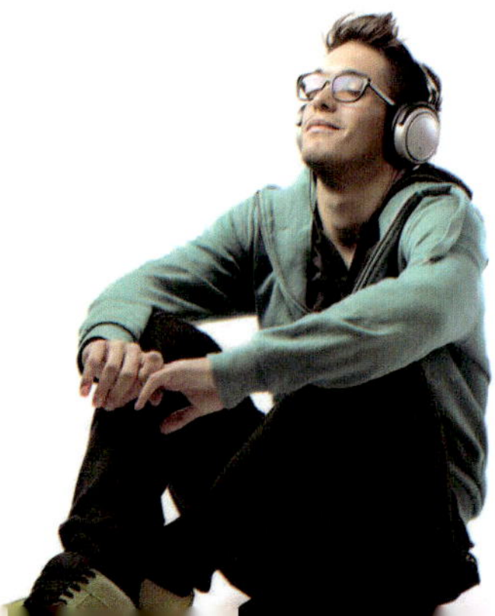

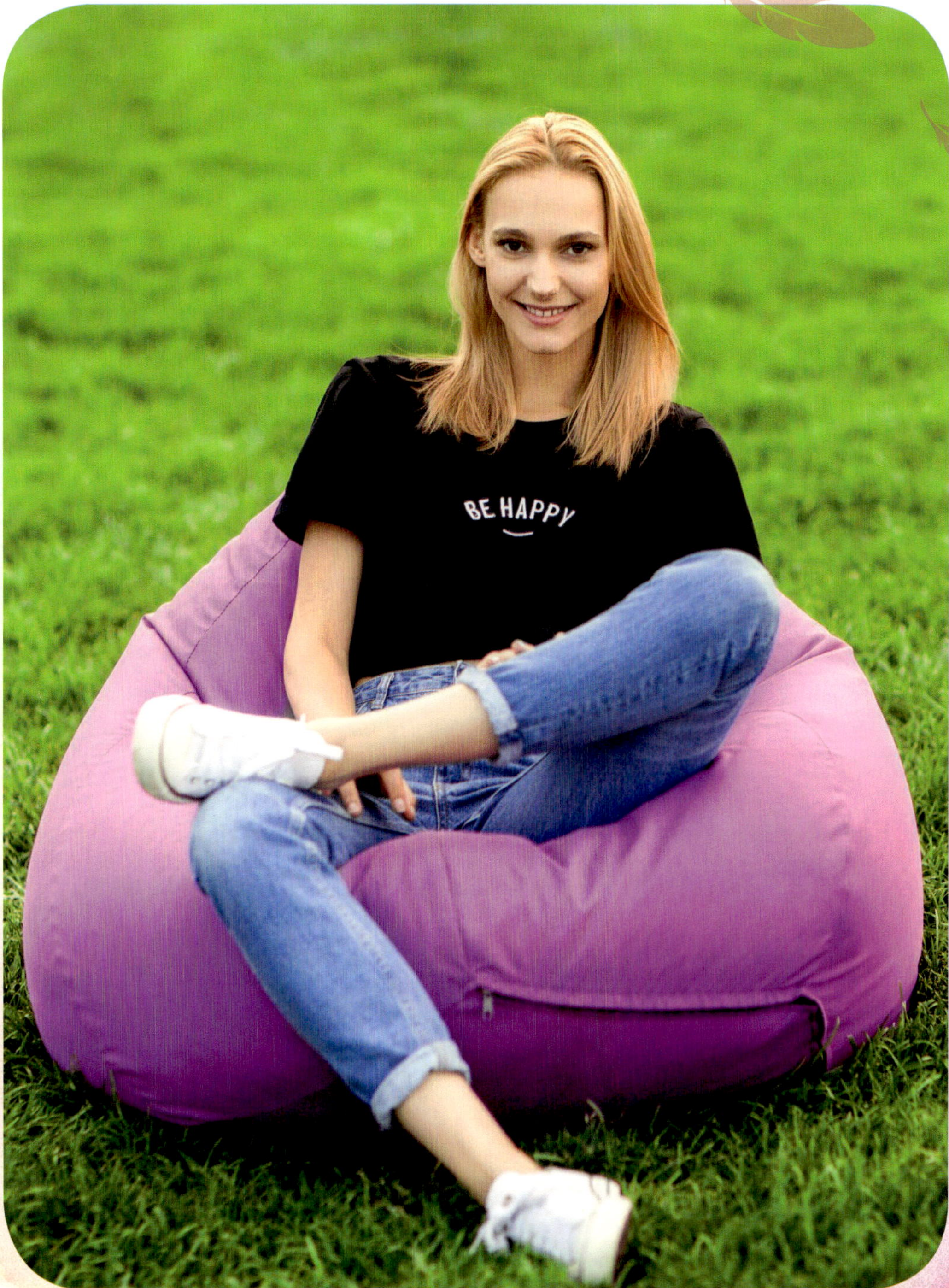
BE HAPPY

CHAPTER FIVE
Use Your Imagination

Sometimes, we need to go on a vacation. But that's not always an easy option. Instead, you can use your **imagination**. Imagination is the mind's ability to be creative.

Pretend you're somewhere else. Imagine you're somewhere calm and peaceful. This could be a beach. It could be a mountaintop. It could be a forest. Pick somewhere that makes you happy.

Create a **script**. A script is a set of written instructions. This will help you imagine your special place. Describe sensory details. Answer these questions: What do you see? What do you hear? What do you feel? What do you taste? What do you touch?

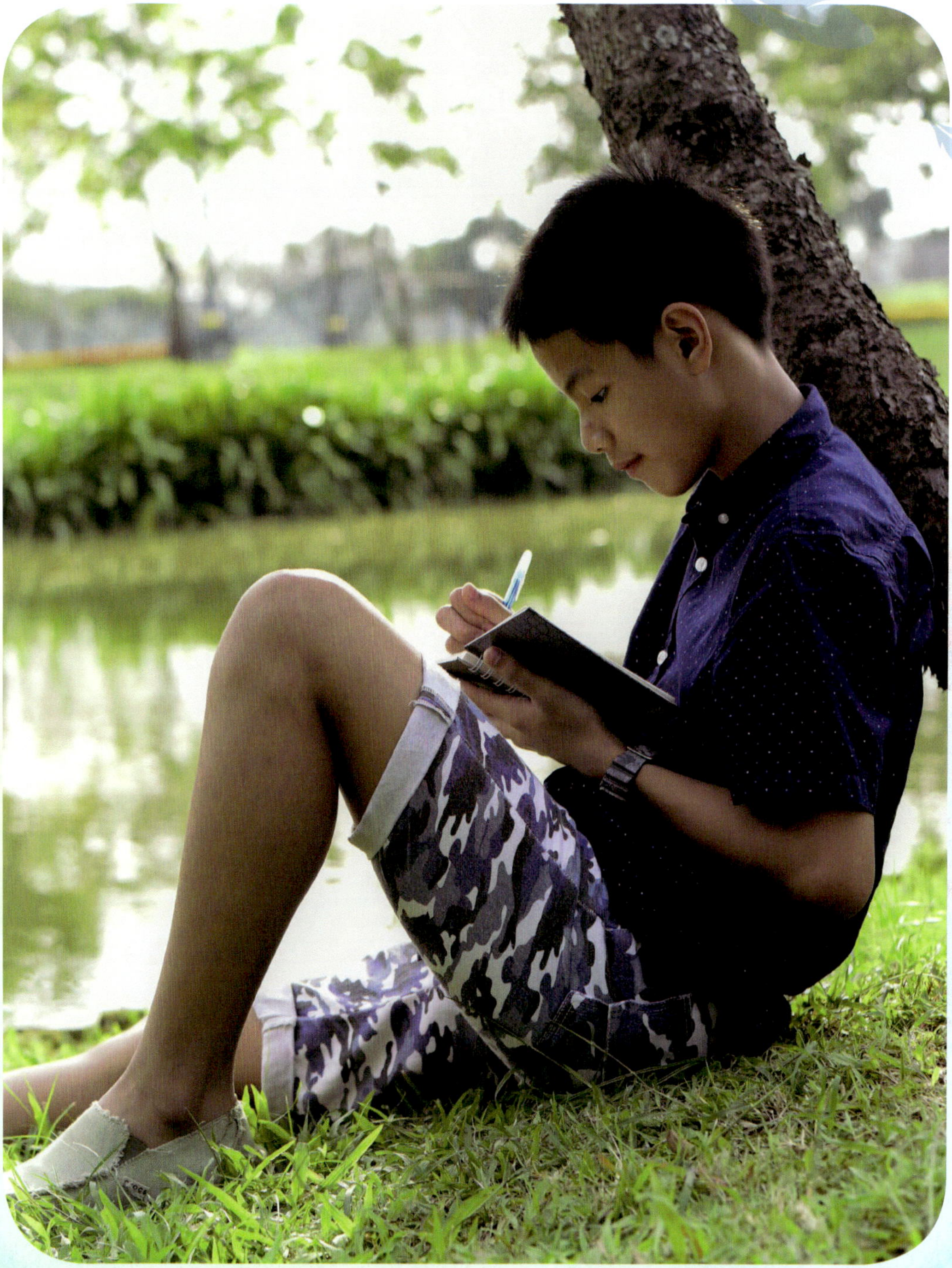

Tip: Journal your feelings. Get it all out on paper.

Imagine walking to your special place. Write out the path you'll take. This will help get you there slowly. This will let you form the image in your mind.

Record your script. Talk in a calm voice. Add details slowly. Include sounds from your special place.

Find a relaxing place. Sit or lie down. Be comfortable. Close your eyes. Take a few deep breaths. Picture your special place in your mind. Play your recording. Remember to breathe slowly. Feel the calm.

Imagine walking back on the path. Count to 3. Open your eyes.

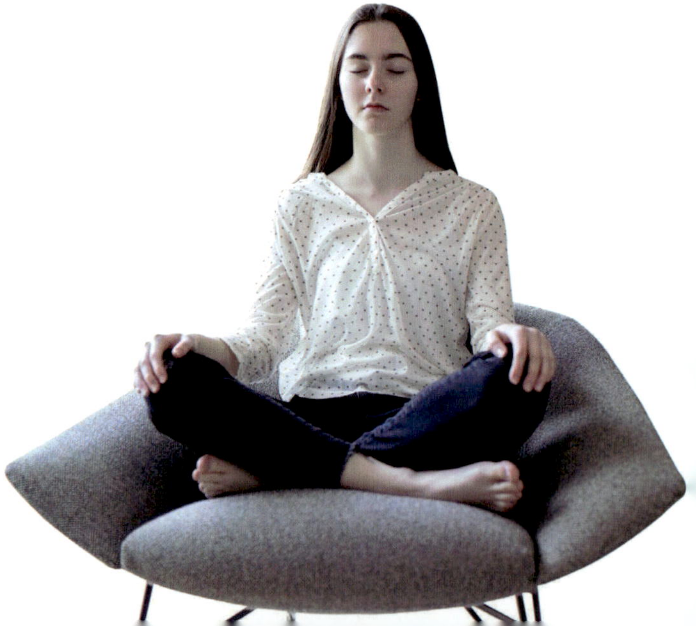

Tip: Create your own calming chair. When you need to calm down, sit in the chair. Don't get up until you feel at peace.

Fun Fact

Petting dogs is calming. It releases stress. It lowers your heart rate. It lowers your blood pressure. It lowers fears. Petting dogs connects people to the present. Dogs have helped college students. College students study a lot. They have to take many tests. Finals are the most important tests. They're the last tests of a class. During finals, college students get really stressed. They have a hard time remembering what they learned. There are programs that bring dogs to college students. These programs train dogs. They send service dogs to people who need help. Students line up to pet dogs. They pet dogs for about 10 minutes. They feel better. Petting the dogs clears their head. It makes them forget about their worries. It helps them focus. These service dogs also help senior citizens, war veterans, and people with special needs.

CHAPTER SIX
Make Your Own Stress Ball

Doing work can be calming. Heavy work means moving the body against heavy **resistance**. Resistance is a force. It's a push and pull. This activates muscles.

Make your own stress ball. Stress balls are things that can be squeezed.

- Blow into a balloon. Stretch it out a bit.
- Stick a **funnel** into the balloon. Funnels are tubes. They guide things into small openings.
- Add rice, flour, sand, or beans. Or add baking soda or hair conditioner. Another option is to use toothpaste.
- Remove the funnel. Let out as much air as you can.
- Tie the balloon tightly.
- Snip off the extra rubber.

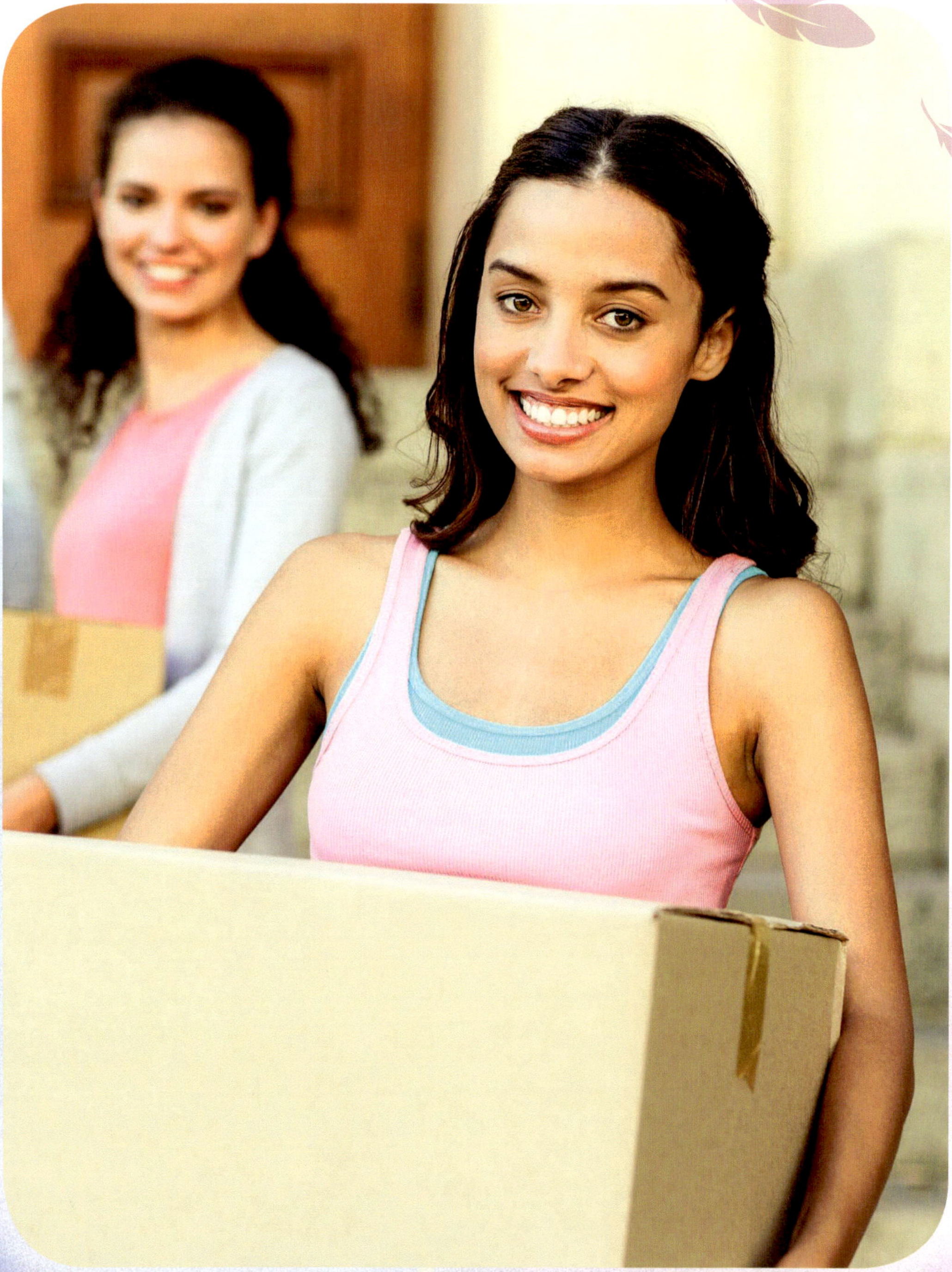

Tip: Do easy heavy-work activities such as moving chairs or desks, carrying books, and holding open heavy doors.

Here are some tips for making the stress balls:

- Get some **mesh**. Mesh is like a net. Wrap the mesh around the balloon. When you squeeze it, parts of the balloon will push through the mesh. This will create an interesting texture.
- Make **emoji** stress balls. Emojis are small pictures of **emotions**. Create a different feeling for each ball using markers. Squeeze the ball with the emotion you're feeling. Change the balls as you calm down.

Do this "tense and relax" activity:

- Hold a stress ball in your hand.
- Bring your shoulders to your ears.
- Count to 5 and relax. Repeat this until you're calm.

Tip: Take a warm bath. Add bubbles or bath salts.

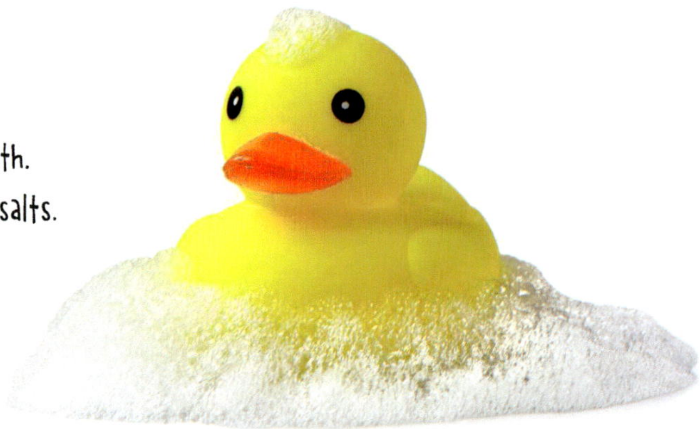

Spotlight Biography

Drinking tea is a great way to calm down. According to a legend, Emperor Shen Nung discovered tea. He rested under a camellia tree. He boiled water to drink. He did this to clean the water. Dried leaves from the tree blew into his water. They mixed in with the water. This made a nice smell. Shen Nung took a sip. He loved the taste. He felt better after drinking it. This happened in 2732 BCE. Shen Nung was from Yunnan, China. Yunnan is in southwestern China. It's the birthplace of tea. Shen Nung's name means "divine farmer." Divine means godly. Shen Nung taught ancient Chinese people how to farm. He taught them how to make medicines from plants. At first, tea was used as medicine. The Chinese have been drinking tea for thousands of years. The first records of tea were found in China.

HOST YOUR OWN MINDFULNESS EVENT!

Feeling riled up? Are you juggling too many things at once? Are you feeling on edge? This might be the best time to host your own mindfulness event! Host a "Be Calm" Party!

STEP ONE: Figure out where you can host your party. You'll need space to spread out.

STEP TWO: Make invitations—and get creative! Ask a friend to help you. Send out the invitations.

STEP THREE: Plan your activities and get supplies.

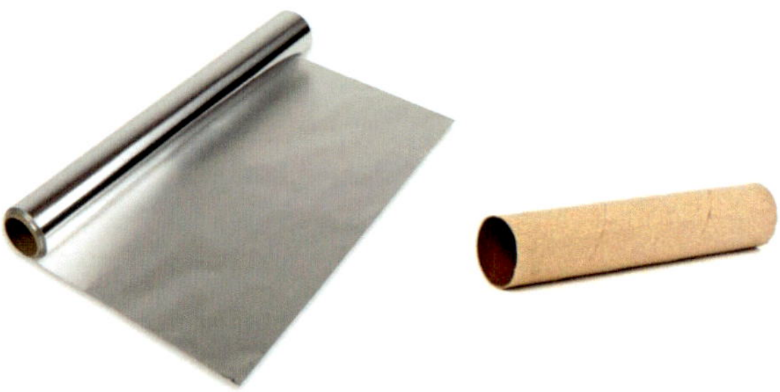

Sticky Hands!

- Tell everyone to imagine they have sticky hands.
- Ask everyone to push their hands together really, really hard. Make sure fingers and palms match up.
- Count out loud to 20.
- Tell everyone to slowly let their hands come apart. Tell them to feel the "stickiness."
- Repeat until everyone feels calm.

Rain Stick Magic!

- Get a plastic wrap tube. Or use a paper towel roll. (Thick cardboard is better.)
- Push or hammer thumbtacks into the tube. (Adding more tacks is better.)
- Wrap foil around the tube, leaving extra foil at both ends.
- Stuff the extra foil into one end of the tube. Leave the other end open.
- Pour rice or beans into the tube.
- Stuff the extra foil into the open end, to close it.
- Decorate your rain stick.
- Tip it to make noise that sounds like rain. Listen to rice or beans fall from one end to the other. Do this until everyone is calm.

Paint It Out!

- Get a plastic shower curtain. Put it on the ground. (Do this outside. Be out in nature.)
- Add shaving cream to the curtain. (Add food coloring dyes if you want colors.)
- Use your hands. Spread out the shaving cream. Paint until you're calm. Push all your worries away.

GLOSSARY

anxious (ANGK-shuhs) extreme worry

channel (CHAN-uhl) to guide or direct

doodling (DOO-duhl-ing) scribbling or drawing

emoji (ih-MOH-jee) a digital image representing an emotion or feeling

emotions (ih-MOH-shuhnz) feelings

funnel (FUHN-uhl) tube used to guide things into a small opening

hobby (HAH-bee) activity done for fun

imagination (ih-maj-uh-NAY-shuhn) mind's ability to be creative, make-believe

massage (muh-SAHZH) rubbing of muscles to relieve pain

mesh (MESH) netting

mindful (MINDE-ful) focusing one's awareness on the present moment to center the mind, body, and soul

panic (PAN-ik) to feel sudden and extreme fear or worry

pinwheel (PIN-weel) stick with a colored wheel that twirls or spins in the wind

resistance (rih-ZIS-tuhns) force involving push and pull

script (SKRIPT) set of written instructions

senses (SENS-iz) sight, hearing, smell, taste, and touch

stressed (STREST) too much pressure and tension

INDEX

About the Author

Dr. Virginia Loh-Hagan is an author, university professor, and former classroom teacher. She's only calm when sleeping. She lives in San Diego with her very tall husband and very naughty dogs. To learn more about her, visit www.virginialoh.com.